e

D1340192

RAY

Please renew/return items by last date
shown. Please call the number below:

Renewals and enquiries: 0300 1234049

Textphone for hearing or
speech impaired users: 01992 555506

www.hertfordshire.gov.uk/libraries   Hertfordshire
L32

Moly Publishing

johnmolyneux.com

52 948 155 2

First published 2019 in the United Kingdom by Moly Publishing

ISBN 978-1-9161271-0-4 (print)
ISBN 978-1-9161271-1-1 (ebook)

Copyright © 2019 John Molyneux, MolyFit Ltd
Reprinted with minor amendments 2019

The author asserts his moral right to be identified as the author of this book. All rights reserved. No part of this publication may be reproduced, stored in a retrieval system, distributed or transmitted, in any form or by any means, without the prior permission in writing of the publisher or as expressly permitted by law.

A catalogue record for this book is available from the British Library
Printed in the United Kingdom

Cover design by Ken Leeder
Photographs by Simon Gill
Illustrations by Duncan Bullimore
Design and layout by Daisy Editorial

Disclaimer

This book is not intended as a substitute for professional medical advice. The reader is advised to consult an appropriate healthcare professional regarding all aspects of individual health care. The author assumes no responsibility for loss or damage caused directly or indirectly by the use of information contained in this book. Individuals who suffer from any disease or are recovering from injury should consult with their doctor regarding the advisability of undertaking any of the exercises suggested in this book. The author disclaims any liability incurred from the use or application of the contents of this book.

Contents

Acknowledgements

I am very fortunate to be blessed with many great and supportive people in my life.

Writing the book was the easy part, but it wouldn't have been anything other than a project sitting in my laptop if it wasn't for all the people that I am privileged to call friends. I would especially like to thank Daniel Barnett for giving me the encouragement and direction to turn my thoughts into a book, Lyndy Katz, my lovely model, for agreeing to be photographed and Simon Gill for taking such great shots.

Photography
Simon Gill

Cover
Ken Leeder

About the Author

John Molyneux has over 20 years' experience as a qualified and accredited sports therapist. He has developed a skill and passion for bringing exercise to those who struggle to maintain a regime or to exercise at all. He has particular expertise in working with age-related barriers, beginning with a gentle and appropriate introduction to exercise and gradually developing ability and confidence.

John firmly believes that exercise is accessible to anyone regardless of their age, ability or physical restrictions. This book is the product of his experience and is an easy-to-use guide for anyone who wants to acquire an exercise routine independently.

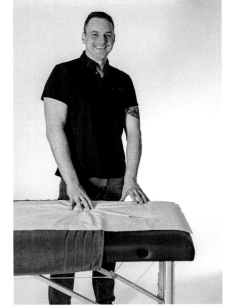

Living well in later life

I have been a sports therapist for 20 years. A sports therapist works with muscles. The work can be dealing with anything from regular muscle pain all the way through to sports injuries. My clients, the people I work for, range from the age of 8 to 98 and include people from all walks of life.

I love my job, and the human body fascinates me. I decided to write this book out of frustration. Every day I come across injuries and problems that could have been avoided. Problems that, if recognised and dealt with earlier, would not have occurred or become so severe.

This book is written with that in mind, to show you how to avoid such problems and make sure that your life is as pain free as possible. Why should you miss out on so many wonderful experiences when maybe, with a little effort and dedication, you could start to live like you remember? It just takes consistency, time and patience.

Now let's get started. Let's build a better you and get you feeling like you used to.

Let's get started

If you don't use them, how do you know that they don't work?

Your body can carry a lot of issues before you realise that there is a problem. Knots, muscle fibres stuck together, tension and stiffness can all live inside you without you realising that they are there. Ever had that pain in your shoulder or neck that just came out of nowhere and was agony for a few weeks? That would have been there building up, growing for months, the muscles getting tighter and tighter until, ahh, pain. It didn't need to get to this, and you could have prevented it altogether. All you needed to do was to be more in touch with your body, recognise the symptoms and fix it. It's easy to do when you know how, but like everything in life, knowledge is power.

Over time, your body develops habits. To see this in action just look at the way you drive, the way you sit in your favourite chair or the way you stand when you are talking to someone. These habits become repeated actions. You do them again and again, and eventually the muscles shorten and tighten. This tightness puts extra stress on your ligaments and joints, which in time can lead to other problems such as wear and tear and arthritis. If you can keep your muscles happy, and minimise their stress, this will help in keeping your bones and joints happy and in their correct position, reducing unnatural wear and tear because everything is sitting where it's meant to be.

Before we start working out what's wrong, let's do a little test.

▶ I want you to stand tall. By this I mean stand up straight. Try to relax your shoulders, and put them where you think they should be.
▶ Take in slow, controlled, regular breaths, in through your nose and out through your mouth.
▶ Now stand with your feet hip distance apart. Look straight ahead and walk on the spot. Don't lift your feet too high. Try to make the action feel as natural as possible.
▶ Do this for one minute continuously and FEEL. Try to take your mind into your body and feel what is going on.

If I were with you, I would be able to see what is going on in your body and help you understand it, but you will have to do the observation yourself. I have found that when people concentrate too hard, they stop breathing, so make sure you breathe, then consider these questions and note anything else you feel.

▶ What are your arms doing? Are they motionless or moving?
▶ Where do you feel tight?
▶ Are you managing to stay on one spot?
▶ Is there pain in your back?
▶ Is one leg working better than the other?

There are so many things you could look out for. I will help you to explore all of these in time, but for now just walk. Walk on the spot for a minute and feel.

Now the minute is over, take a moment to think. Listen to your body. What is it telling you? What was the most important thing you took from that exercise? Did everything feel ok or was there something niggling that perhaps shouldn't have been? You can learn an awful amount from just one minute of simple exercise, listening to your body.

When I take on a new client, the first thing they often say to me after a session is, "Well, that never used to hurt before". Well, of course it didn't, because they never used it and didn't know there was as problem. Our lives are so busy that we become detached from ourselves. We stop listening and stop feeling. It's now time to reverse that and take back control. Time to stop ignoring the problems and do something about them.

Posture

Posture is the way you carry yourself. It's the position in which you hold your body either sitting or standing. It's by far my biggest gripe. I say this because, if you can get your posture right, most things will then fall into place. We are not told how to walk, how to run, how to stand or how to sit; we have just done it, learnt it ourselves. I always say that if this was taught in schools, as part of the national curriculum, I would have far fewer clients.

There are four types of postural alignment. If you look at the diagram on the next page you can see how you are meant to stand and probably how you actually stand.

Test it out. Stand side on to a mirror and take a photo, then see which type you are. Keep the photo as you will need it for later on.

Now let's see what condition your posture is in.

► Stand with your back against a wall.
► Place your heels, bottom, shoulders and head against the wall at the same time and hold that position for 30 seconds.
► As in the first exercise, breathe and listen to your body.

Four types of posture

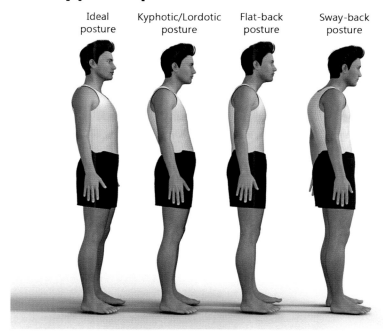

Ideal posture   Kyphotic/Lordotic posture   Flat-back posture   Sway-back posture

► Are you able to stand there quite comfortably, or is 30 seconds feeling like a long time?
► Is there a strain in your neck where you are forcing your head back?
► Are you arching your lower back trying to get your shoulders into position?

If everything is ok then that position should feel absolutely comfortable. If it's not then we have work to do.

If you are going to improve your posture then you should definitely start with your spine. In my eyes, the most important component in total body health is maintaining a neutral lumbar spine. Or in other words, sorting out your lower back! Through bad posture, your lower back is where you hold all the tension and stress built up in your body during the day. It keeps building up until, one day, it simply can't cope any more. Your muscles go into spasm, your hips go out of alignment or you damage a disc.

Basically, things are not in the position they are meant to be in and something has to give.

First of all, you have to work out what is a neutral lower spine. If you look at the diagram you can clearly see what is right and what is not.

If it's right, great; everything works as it should. If it's not then all your body weight is passing though your lower back, and that is what gets you into trouble. Body weight should pass naturally through your core, thighs and feet, not your back.

Let's start working at taking the pressure out of your back to where it should go. For this you need to lie on the floor. If you feel uncomfortable doing this or are worried that you won't make it back up, lie on your bed and do it there.

▸ Lie on your back with your knees bent and feet flat on the floor (see diagram).
▸ Make sure the space is even between your feet and legs up to your thighs.
▸ Rest your arms down straight at your sides.
▸ Relax your body, take in a few deep breaths, always in through your nose and out through your mouth.

Feel the air passing through your body, your chest expanding to bring it in and your stomach (diaphragm) pushing it out. Allow your shoulders, neck and back to rest on the floor without effort.

If this feels too uncomfortable then place a small cushion under your head for a little support. Try to feel your rib cage relaxing, releasing to the floor. Your lower back should feel comfortable. It should not be too arched and it should not be too flat. It should be just right. If you are in the correct position then you shouldn't feel your lower back at all. Look at the diagram and try to imagine yourself in that position.

Now just lie there and breathe. Try to picture what your body should be doing and try to feel that your lower back is in the correct position. This is a neutral lower spine. Not too arched, not too flat, just right. I'm not expecting you to master it straight away. It will take time and practice. Try it a few times, and when you feel ready and think you have got it then you probably have. The next step is putting it into practice with movement in everyday life.

⮩ Lie on floor, knees bent

Maintain a neutral spine

Try to relax your neck, shoulders and back

Keep your knees at 45 degrees

Feet and legs even space apart

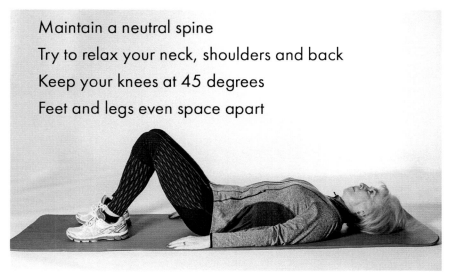

3

Core work

I think of the core as the starting point of any body action. Your core is responsible for holding everything in place when you use your body. This involves many muscles, from those deep inside to the muscles you can see on the surface. At this stage, you don't need to understand all of these muscles. All I want is for you to understand how to engage your core and, in doing so, protect your back.

Let's go back to the previous exercise. Lie down on the floor or your bed with your knees bent and feet flat. Put your lower back into the neutral position. Remember, not too arched and not too flat. When you are happy your spine is neutral, try the following exercise.

- ▶ Keeping your heels down, lift your toes off the floor.
- ▶ Now, gently try to raise your heels off the floor. Only lift them a little, not too high.
- ▶ You should feel your lower back arching up and pressure going into your spine.

This is what you don't want to happen. Your body can be lazy and will always find the easiest way to do something. In this example, your back has taken over and you are putting all the weight of the effort into your back. This is what happens throughout the whole day without you even realising. You do an action, use your back instead of your core and eventually... a bad back.

Now let's do it right. Get yourself into the neutral spine position. Heels down, toes off the floor.

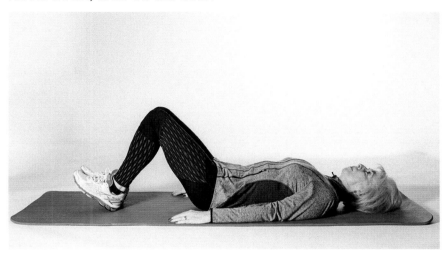

Take in some slow, deep breaths and gently pull in your navel. Don't pull too much. If you try too hard, you may pull a muscle and then there will be no exercise for you for several weeks. Pull in your navel just enough to feel the muscles behind it working. You should feel the muscles gently activating, not straining or pulling.

Now, with those muscles engaged, gently pull the force up towards your chin.

Think about what you can feel. You should feel your internal muscles tucking in.

Try to hold that position for 10 seconds, but remember to keep breathing. One of the core muscles is your diaphragm so it's quite normal to hold everything in during this exercise and forget to breathe!

Try this five times, holding for 10 seconds each time. The exercise should feel gentle and natural with no pain or discomfort. When you are doing this, you should feel no movement in your lower back. Your spine should be neutral and you should only feel the muscles you are trying to activate. You are trying to isolate your core.

If you are happy with this and feel that you can isolate your core without affecting your back, let's put it into practice!

Core strengthening exercises

Single leg raise with bent knee

▸ Lie on your back, knees bent, feet flat on the floor with your arms by your side.
▸ As before, adopt a neutral spine and engage your core. Try not to strain; pull in just enough to feel the muscles.
▸ Now, raise your toes on one leg, keeping the heel on the floor.
▸ Making sure you keep your core switched on, raise the heel slightly off the floor, about the height of a closed fist.
▸ Repeat this action five times with the first leg, making sure your spine stays neutral. Then repeat with the other leg.

When doing this, keep your knee in the same position so the exercise comes from your hip.

➲ Single/double leg raise with bent knee

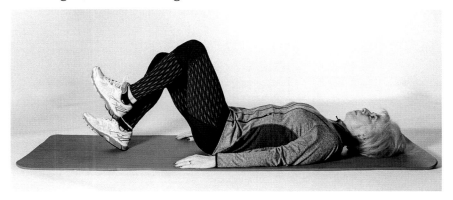

If you are doing the exercise correctly, you will feel your lower back hasn't moved. You will also feel your core, thigh and hip muscles working.

If you haven't quite mastered it, you will feel it in your back and you will feel your pelvis tilting towards the leg you are lifting.

If you are happy with this then try the same exercise with both legs raised. This is tougher as you are doubling the workload and lifting the weight of both your legs through your core.

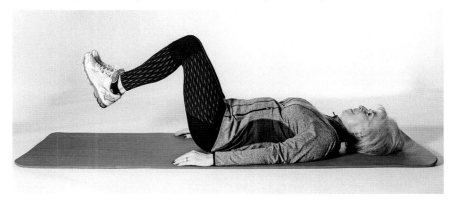

This exercise is really hard to master. If you can do this then it's a massive achievement. It's a complicated action to get right because you have to activate your core to stabilise the action. The whole weight of your legs is passing through your core.

If you can do it, let's move on to putting it in place with the rest of your body. If you're not quite there yet, don't worry. With a little practice, you'll have it in no time.

Standing with engaged core

Earlier on, you looked at a diagram of correct posture and took a photo of yourself. I want you to take another, this time with your core switched on.

Stand side on to the mirror. Relax your shoulders and soften your knees. Now think about your neutral spine and try to put it into the same position as when you were on the floor. Engage your core. Gently pull in your navel and imagine drawing it up to your chin. Not too much, just enough to feel the muscles working. Now hold that position for a few seconds, remembering to breathe.

When you are ready, take a photo. Compare it with the first one you took. You may be amazed by what you see!

Let's add some movement.

Stand with your feet hip distance apart and with a neutral spine, then engage your core.

Try to walk on the spot. Don't use a stiff or rigid movement. Make it feel natural. If it doesn't, then you are simply trying too hard.

Relax your shoulders and swing your arms. Try doing this for one minute, constantly checking to see if your core is still on. If it is, you will feel it. The exercise should feel completely different to before.

You should feel taller, more open and relaxed. Your body should feel lighter and not fighting you, as it may have felt before.

➲ Standing with engaged core

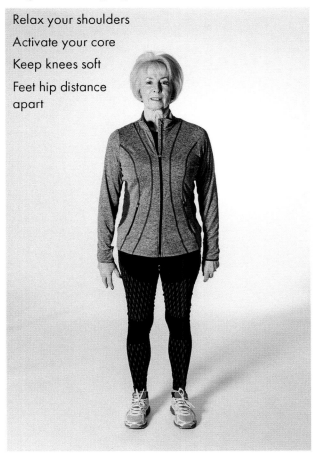

Relax your shoulders

Activate your core

Keep knees soft

Feet hip distance apart

Now add the icing on the cake and complete your transformation. Start walking on the spot as before, only this time open your chest. You will feel your shoulders lifting and your chest expanding. Don't force it; let it be a natural movement. Keeping your chest open is very important, and this is why.

The seven shoulder joint movements

The shoulder is a ball-and-socket joint, which gives it a massive range of movement – the most of any joint type in your body. The problem with this huge range of movement is that when the muscles around your shoulder become tight, the joint can pull towards them. The more range of movement in the joint, the more susceptible it becomes to muscular imbalance.

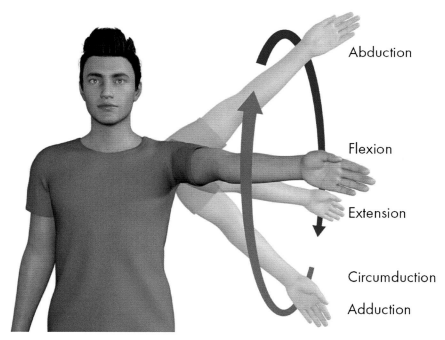

Abduction

Flexion

Extension

Circumduction

Adduction

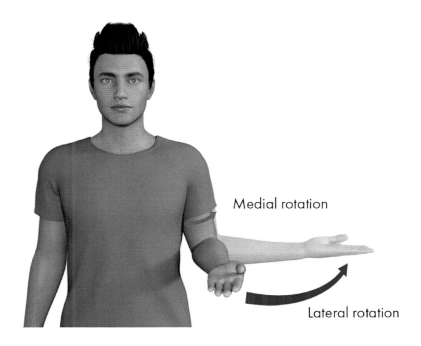

Medial rotation

Lateral rotation

An everyday example of how muscular imbalance can happen is using your computer.

Firstly, there is no way that you will sit in front of it with your core always on. Most of the time you will slouch. There is just too much else going on to be constantly aware of how you are sitting. As you slouch, your body slumps forward, putting pressure on your back. Your shoulders move forward, tightening your chest. Then your shoulders are no longer sitting in their correct position, which puts more pressure on your neck and upper back.

You can avoid all this from happening by opening your chest, trying to have your core on more often and taking little breaks from your desk every 20 minutes to reset your body position.

Let's do a little test to show you what I mean. Stand up and switch on your core, with a neutral spine and open chest. With one hand, gently pull down on the other by the wrist. You should feel a gentle pull in your shoulder and down your arm. Now do the same but without your core on or your chest open. The pull you feel this time will have shifted to your neck. This is because, without an open chest, your shoulders have dropped forward and in doing so are pulling on your neck muscles.

Basically, if all your muscles are in the right place, everything tends to work as it should. When they are not, you create imbalance and tension in your body, which leads to muscles in the wrong place, acting in the wrong way. By the end of this book, hopefully you will be back in touch with your body and all this will start to make sense.

Going for a walk

Now you are going to put what you have learnt so far into practice. I want you to go for a short walk, anything from 5 to 20 minutes.

Before you do that, however, I want to add in an extra consideration. When you are walking, walk heel to toe. Concentrate on each foot to make sure that you strike the ground with your heel first.

Feel the pressure roll towards the balls of your feet then push off with your toes.

This little exercise makes sure your muscles are used effectively and efficiently, putting less tension in them and using less energy.

Before you start walking, here is your checklist.

- ▸ Maintain a neutral spine.
- ▸ Gently activate your core.
- ▸ Open your chest and relax your shoulders.
- ▸ Swing your arms.
- ▸ Walk heel to toe.
- ▸ Take deep, regular breaths, in through your nose and out through your mouth.

I know this is a lot to remember, but once you have got it, walking will feel so much easier.

Now go for that walk.

⊃ Balls of feet

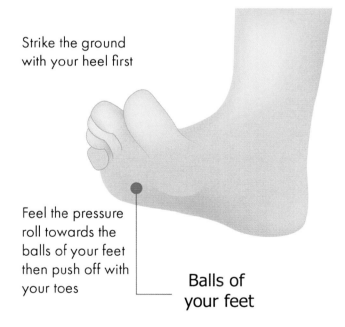

Strike the ground with your heel first

Feel the pressure roll towards the balls of your feet then push off with your toes

Balls of your feet

⋏ ⋏ ⋏

So how did it feel? Did you manage to keep your core on the whole time, and did you remember to breathe? Did your back feel ok? Were your thighs aching? Could you feel any muscles pulling that you thought should not have? I bet it felt robotic and wooden, completely unnatural. This is because you have just started to make a dent in all your body's bad habits. You have asked it to do what it should be doing and tried to stop it from doing what it wants. It will put up a bit of a fight. But persevere: the end result will be worth it.

In the next part of the book you will learn how to recognise what your body is telling you. You will learn how to look out for the signs that you have unwanted tension and muscular imbalances, and you will learn how to deal with them. In the meantime, practice going on short walks using the checklist above. When you are more familiar with the technique, start thinking about what else you can feel as you walk. Make a note of those little niggles and aches that should not be there so you can deal with them later.

4

Starting to exercise

Let's start strengthening and stretching your muscles. Here you will learn how to look out for problems in your body and deal with them accordingly. The main problems you will be looking out for are weakness and imbalance. If you can target them early enough, it will stop them from becoming habits. A habit is harder to treat and can lead to chronic issues if left to get worse.

The older you get, the faster your muscles waste away, especially with underuse. This is called atrophy. From birth until your thirties, your muscles grow stronger. After that, you start to lose muscle mass and function. This will happen even if you stay active, so if you are not active, the effect will be worse. If you exercise and keep your muscles as strong as possible, this will help reduce frailty and the possibility of falls and other damage.

The best form of exercise for this is strength training, and the best piece of equipment for that is you! Using your body weight for exercise strengthens your muscles and also helps retain bone density.

If your bones and muscles are strong and in good working order, it will help prevent unwanted outcomes such as a broken hip after a fall because you didn't pick your feet up enough or because you tripped on the kerb, or a fall down the stairs because your legs gave way due to weakness.

All the following exercises just need you, no fancy equipment or expensive gym membership. The hardest thing about exercise is getting off your chair and doing it – finding the motivation. You will only exercise effectively if you want to do it; but, believe me, just a few minutes a day can have a dramatic impact on the rest of your life.

So, let's get started and make sure the rest of your life is full and active and not full of limitations, with you sitting your days out on your favourite chair.

The door hinge

The first exercise I want you to do is called the door hinge. This is a great all-rounder and will really give you an idea of what is tight in your body and needs your attention. The door hinge is one of my favourite exercises.

Everyday life makes us tight and puts a strain on our body. This is a great exercise to press the reset button after a day of driving a car, or sitting in traffic, or carrying heavy bags of shopping.

It really does help shake off all the tension and takes out those knots that are just waiting to form.

Whether you think you need it or not, I definitely recommend getting this exercise into your daily routine. It's a great all-round preventative, helping to ease the strain in so many muscles.

Muscles stretched in the door hinge

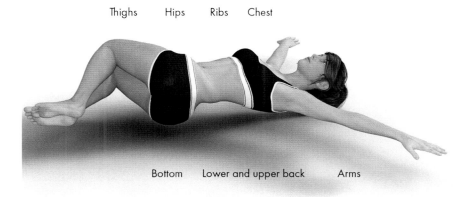

Thighs Hips Ribs Chest

Bottom   Lower and upper back   Arms

For this exercise you will need a pillow.

- ► Lie on your side with your knees bent and your head on the pillow for support. Place your arms straight out in front of you, palms together.
- ► Now, with your legs pressed together and fixed on the floor, but allowing your top half to twist round, move your top arm up and over, all the way to the floor behind you (or as far as you can comfortably reach). As you do so, let your eyes follow your fingertips. Do the action slowly and with control. If you rush, you may pull that tight muscle that has been hiding.
- ► As soon as the back on your hand hits the floor (or reaches your comfort point), take a breath and bring your arm back to the starting position.

Do this 10 times on each side. If you are struggling to reach the floor, don't push too hard. Just try to go a little further each time. Unless there is a real problem, you should be able to reach the floor by the tenth time.

You will feel the stretch of this exercise in the area that is tight. The usual suspects are your chest, arms, hips, ribs or lower back. Make a note of where you feel the tension pulling. You'll stretch it out later on.

➲ The door hinge

Feet and legs stay together

Keep arms straight

Knees bent

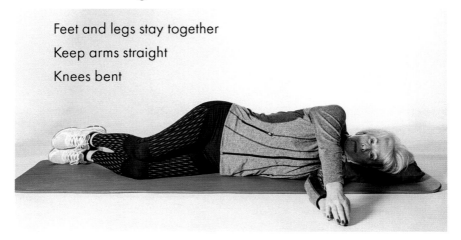

Eyes follow fingertips

Feet and legs stay together

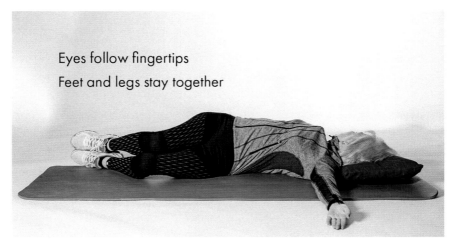

The chest stretch

A tight chest will pull your shoulders forward, put pressure on your neck and back and make it really difficult to maintain your core. The pectoral muscles in your chest are strong and very powerful. To give you an idea of their strength, they can be trained to lift your own body weight! Pretty much everybody has tight chest muscles, so they really need looking after to work well. When tight, they contribute to bad posture and can restrict your breathing. The pecs attach to your rib cage, so if they are tight, your ribs can't expand to their full potential, limiting the amount of air going into your lungs in deep breathing.

Let's start loosening off those pecs.

➲ Chest stretch

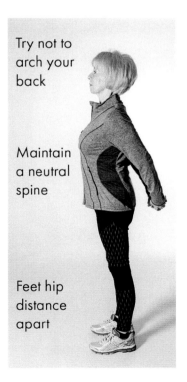

Try not to arch your back

Maintain a neutral spine

Feet hip distance apart

- ▸ Stand tall with a neutral spine and your feet hip distance apart.
- ▸ Open your chest and relax your shoulders. Activate your core.
- ▸ With straight arms, interlock your fingers behind you. Push your arms up while pulling your shoulder blades together.
- ▸ Stop and hold the stretch when you feel your chest opening and your arms won't go up any further.
- ▸ Hold for 20 seconds, taking in big breaths. Breathe in through your nose and out through your mouth. Keep looking forward, trying not to bend your neck.

5

Lower back

Everyone experiences some degree of lower back pain at some time. As I mentioned earlier, a lot of that can be attributed to a lack of correct posture. When your posture is poor, your spine is not neutral and your body weight goes into your lower back. Let's first do a stretch to see how flexible your spine is.

The cat stretch

Gently get down onto the floor on your hands and knees. With your arms and legs parallel, an equal distance apart, pull your belly in and slowly round up through your spine, lower back, shoulders and neck, arching your spine towards the ceiling. Gently let your head drop. Hold this stretch for 30 seconds, and remember to breathe.

The main area you should feel this in is your back. As you arch up you should feel the muscles pulling either side of your spine. It should feel comfortable, not painful. If you feel pain, stop, take a breath and try again. If the pain is still there the second time, stop. When your muscles are tight or in spasm you can't force them, as this will just make it worse.

One tip if you are having difficulty doing this is to warm up your muscles first. When muscles are warm they are more flexible, so you can get much more out of them. Easy ways to do this are by using a heated wheat bag or having a bath for 20 minutes and relaxing. Let your muscles warm up and ease off. When you feel ready, try the cat stretch again. If it doesn't feel better and you are still having trouble, persevere a few more times then, if no better, seek professional advice.

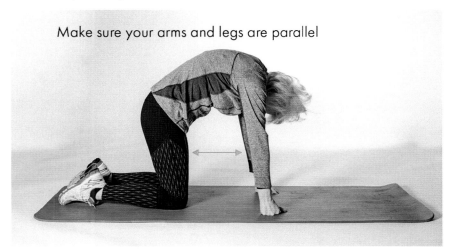

Make sure your arms and legs are parallel

The sacroiliac joint

The sacroiliac joint connects the spine to the pelvis. There are two in your lower back, one each side of the spine just above your tail bone. They support the weight of your entire upper body when you are upright and are important for walking.

First, let's have a look and see what condition your sacroiliac joints are in. Be careful with these exercises and don't force them. If you have an injury in the sacroiliac joint, it's easy to make it worse.

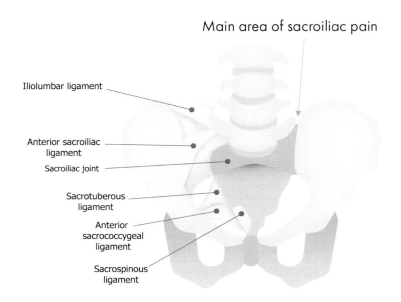

Main area of sacroiliac pain

Iliolumbar ligament

Anterior sacroiliac ligament

Sacroiliac joint

Sacrotuberous ligament

Anterior sacrococcygeal ligament

Sacrospinous ligament

When doing these exercises, you should only feel a stretch, not pain. If you feel pain then stop. The muscles around this area are big and powerful. If they tense up or go into spasm, the result is also big and powerful. You will not be able to stand up straight, walk or sit properly and will experience strong pain in the lower back area, especially just to the side of your spine. If you are experiencing this pain already or something doesn't feel right when you do these exercises then it is definitely worth a trip to see a professional or your doctor.

Knee to chest stretch

Let's start with one of the more gentle sacroiliac joint stretches. I like to start off slowly and carefully. It's better to recognise you have a problem doing a gentle exercise, stop and get it treated than jump into an advanced exercise and cause more injury that will take weeks to get over.

For this exercise you can do one leg at a time or both legs together. I suggest you start with one leg and, if it feels ok, move on to two.

- Lie on your back with your knees bent, feet flat on the floor.
- Take a deep breath in and, as you breathe out, pull your knee towards your chest. Pull with your hands placed on the back of your thigh, not from the knee, as you want to avoid any unnecessary pressure on the knee joint.
- Hold the stretch for 10 seconds and breathe in again as you lower your leg back down.

Repeat with the other leg and continue alternating until you have done it five times on each side. If all feels good then try the same exercise with both legs together, again holding for 10 seconds and repeating five times.

➲ Knee to chest stretch

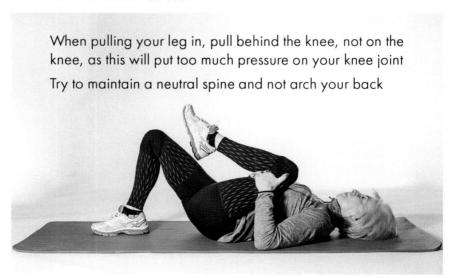

When pulling your leg in, pull behind the knee, not on the knee, as this will put too much pressure on your knee joint

Try to maintain a neutral spine and not arch your back

Legs down to one side

▶ Lie on your back with your knees bent and feet flat on the floor. Make sure your feet are a little distance apart, not touching.
▶ With your arms straight, slightly away from your body, pin your shoulders to the floor. If your shoulders rise when you do this exercise you will not feel the benefit of the stretch in your back.
▶ Gently and slowly, with your legs going in the same direction, let your knees fall down to one side.
▶ When your legs are down as far as they can go, hold the stretch for 30 seconds, then repeat on the other side.

Remember to anchor your body with your arms and shoulders, trying to keep them on the floor. Don't force the stretch; let your legs fall down naturally.

➲ Legs down to one side

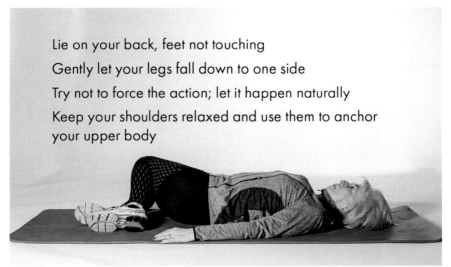

Lie on your back, feet not touching

Gently let your legs fall down to one side

Try not to force the action; let it happen naturally

Keep your shoulders relaxed and use them to anchor your upper body

If that felt good, without pain or discomfort, then you can try to open up your sacroiliac joint a little more with some gentle movement.

Windscreen wipers

► Lie on your back with your knees bent and feet flat on the floor.
► Gently let your knees fall down together to one side. Don't force the movement, but carefully let them fall.
► Hold for a few seconds and then return your knees to the centre, the start position.

Now repeat this on the other side and keep going until you have done it five times on each side.

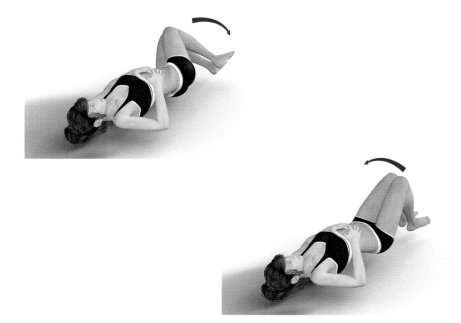

The Superman

This is a lower back strengthening exercise. It's a great exercise as it works the muscles in your lower back while maintaining a neutral spine.

A lot of lower back exercises can be detrimental as they make you hyperextend your back by bending it backwards. If you have a disc problem, or degenerative changes in your spine, that may result in you feeling pain. The Superman exercise, however, should not cause you pain. It's a great way of strengthening your back without aggravating it.

► Lie on your front with your forehead on the floor. Place your arms out in front of you at full stretch and keep your legs long.
► Gently and slowly raise your left arm and right leg a little, just enough to feel them coming off the floor. Keep your arms and legs straight.
► Bring your arm and leg back down and repeat with the right arm and left leg. Do this five times on each side.

Keep your forehead on the floor, and try not to raise it

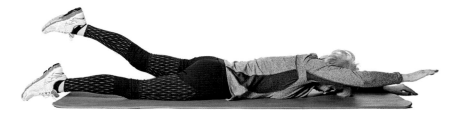

6

Upper back

For this exercise you will need a tea towel and a chair. The type of chair is extremely important. When you sit in a chair to exercise, you want to make sure that your knees are at the same height as your bottom or slightly lower.

If your knees are higher than your bottom, this changes the angle of your hips and lower back and makes it difficult to maintain a neutral spine. A classic example of this is sitting on a sofa. On a nice comfy sofa you will see your knees are much higher than your bottom. Now try to stand up from that position with correct posture and a neutral spine. It just doesn't happen. The only way to do it is to shuffle to the edge of the sofa, sit up straight and push up with your core and thighs.

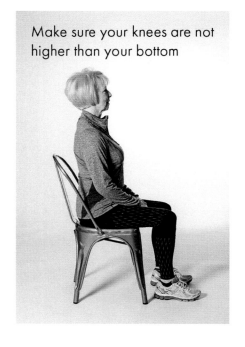

Make sure your knees are not higher than your bottom

Watch people when they stand up from a seated position. Firstly, their hands go on their knees putting unnecessary body weight into the knees, then they lean forward, putting too much body weight into their back. They then push up with a bent back, with their knees turning inwards, and finally straighten up, with all their body weight in their lower back.

➲ Things to avoid when standing from seated

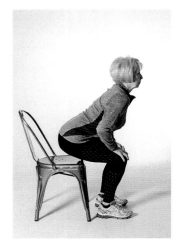

- ► Avoid bending forward and placing your hands on your knees.
- ► Try to stand up with a neutral spine, keeping your bodyweight out of your back and instead using your bottom, thighs and core.

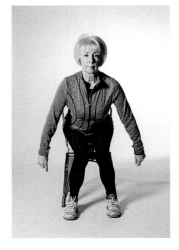

- ► Avoid bringing your knees together.
- ► Keep your knees apart.
- ► Your knee should be over your foot

- ▶ Try to avoid standing using your back
- ▶ Keep your spine neutral and don't lean forward

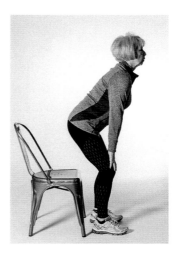

Use the following technique to stand from a sitting position in a way that will strengthen your muscles instead of weakening them.

- ▶ Sit on the chair with your core on and a neutral spine.
- ▶ Place your feet at hip distance apart, toes slightly facing out.
- ▶ Take in a breath.
- ▶ With relaxed shoulders and an open chest, breathe out and push up using your thighs, buttocks and core muscles.

Through this exercise you have strengthened your core, thighs, buttocks, back and hips, as well as your body in general. Before learning this technique, you were at risk of weakening your body and causing imbalances through habit.

Imagine if you had the discipline to stand in this way every time you got up from a chair? By just using this simple technique you are doing a power of good for your body. You are exercising naturally and keeping your muscles strong with minimal effort.

Tea towel pulls

- Sit on a suitable chair that allows your knees to be level with your bottom, with your spine away from the back of the chair.
- Have your feet hip distance apart and your knees bent at a 90-degree angle. This is important because if your feet are pulled back behind your knees, that will engage the back of your thighs, which will pull on your back.
- Now hold the tea towel by each end above your head. Keep it taut but don't pull too hard. Engage your core and make sure your spine is neutral.
- Keep your eyes facing forward and pull the tea towel down behind you to the base of your neck, keeping the towel straight.
- Then pull the towel back up again to the starting position.

If all is well you should have managed to pull the tea towel up and down with ease, working the muscles in your upper back. If you have a tight chest, neck or shoulders, your head may have tilted forward, or you may have felt a pull in your neck or back where you were straining, or your arms wouldn't let you pull down to the base of your neck without a bend in the towel. This is all down to tightness and imbalance in your neck, chest, arms and upper back.

To try to fix the problem, don't do too much at once. If you can't pull the towel down to your neck without it bending or your head dipping, just pull it down to the top of your head. When you can do that, try to pull it down slightly behind your head, and then pull it down to your ears. Do this in stages and eventually your muscles will loosen off, enabling you to pull the tea towel right down to the base of your neck. When you can do this, you will really feel the benefit of your chest opening and stretching, and your shoulders and muscles in your upper back strengthening.

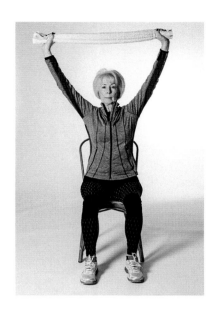 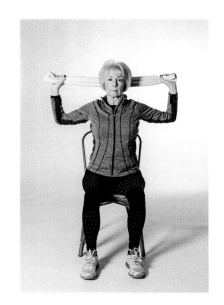

- ▶ Try not to arch your back by maintaining a neutral spine.
- ▶ Keep the towel taut.
- ▶ Only pull down to your neck, no lower.
- ▶ Don't bend or tilt your neck.

Now you are going to stretch the large muscle in your upper back, the trapezius. It's one of the muscles that will play up if you are under stress or have poor posture. It will cause aching or sometimes burning sensations from the top of your neck down to your shoulder blade. When things get really bad, you may even feel

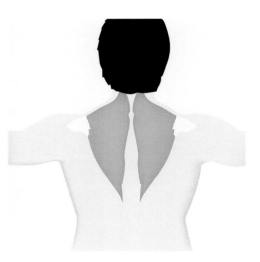

this down your arm. This muscle is easily what I spend most of my day treating with massage. Whether it's down to a tight chest pulling the shoulders forward, bad posture or emotional stress, these factors all affect the trapezius muscle, causing knots and tension. Other common reasons for trapezius tension are holding a phone between your ear and shoulder, carrying a heavy bag, and bra straps that are too tight. All place too much stress on the muscle, which causes it over time to shorten and tense up.

Chin to chest stretch

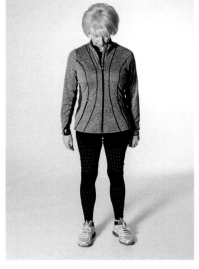

- ▶ Do this exercise sitting down. Sit up straight with your core engaged and a neutral spine. Relax your shoulders and breathe in.
- ▶ As you exhale, slowly bring your head forward, taking your chin towards your neck and down to your chest. You should feel the stretch running from your shoulder blades all the way to the base of your skull.
- ▶ Hold this stretch for 30 seconds. When finished, try not to raise your head up too quickly to avoid dizziness.

Shoulder shrugs

- ▶ Stand up with an engaged core and neutral spine.
- ▶ Pull your shoulders up to your ears. Hold for a few seconds and then gently lower them to a relaxed position.
- ▶ Repeat this 10 times.

If this feels ok, add a roll. Pull your shoulders up to your ears and then roll them back behind you. When they reach their highest point, start to lower them to a relaxed position. Repeat this 10 times.

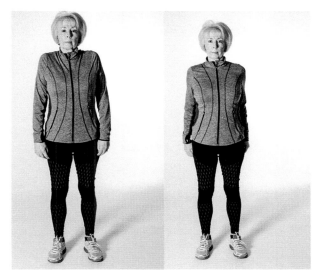

Feet hip distance apart with soft knees

Neutral spine, don't arch your back

Feel the muscles 'crunching' as they loosen

You may feel some crunching or clicking. Don't worry – this is a good thing! You are feeling the knots in the muscles loosening off, relieving the tension. Muscle is a soft tissue. When you touch it, it should feel soft and relaxed. When it's tight it becomes stiff and hard as the fibres shorten. When I'm massaging, this is what I'm looking for, feeling through touch. Sometimes, the muscles get so tight and so hard they actually feel like bone. This is when the massage gets deep and my elbow comes out. The tissue becomes so stiff and knotted that my fingers just haven't got the strength to break it up, so I have to use my body weight, directed through my elbow, to start easing off the tension. When it gets to this stage, I am literally ripping the muscle fibres apart to separate them. It's not a nice massage and I don't like doing it as it causes my clients pain, but it's what needs to be done.

Hug the tree stretch

- ▶ Stand up with your feet hip distance apart, with soft knees and a neutral spine.
- ▶ Imagine that there is a massive tree in front of you with a large trunk and give it a cuddle. Hug it with your fingers clasped together and elbows bent.
- ▶ Feel the trapezius muscles pulling away from each other, pulling outwards away from your spine. Draw that feeling into your shoulders and down your arms.
- ▶ Gently lower head so you are looking at the floor. This will stretch the trapezius further. When you are happy that you can feel an effective stretch, hold it for 30 seconds.

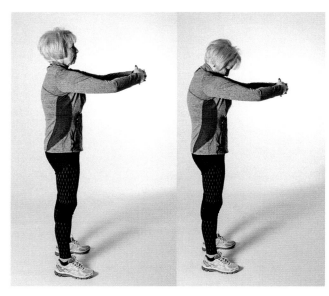

Feel your shoulder blades pulling away from your spine as you stretch

Lower your head to fully stretch the trapezius

7

Hip and bottom

Like the shoulder, the hip joint allows a big range of movement. The muscles around the hip have to cope with a lot of stresses and pressure as the hip supports your bodyweight and the massive force that comes from the large muscles of the leg. The muscles in the hip and bottom are very strong and very powerful. They have to be to keep your hip in place, stopping it from dislocating from the extra movement in the joint. During movement, especially running and jumping, the force on the body multiplies many times and your hip must be able to cope with these forces repeatedly.

When a client of mine points to where their pain is, especially lower back pain, a lot of the time the problem stems from the muscles around the hip and bottom. The pain is 'referred'. In other words, they may feel it in their lower back but the actual cause is the big, powerful muscles of the hip and bottom.

I am constantly working with my clients on the gluteus muscles (the big, powerful muscles of the bottom), the piriformis (a deep muscle that causes many problems) and the iliopsoas (a complex muscle that can be the source of so many niggles and back pain).

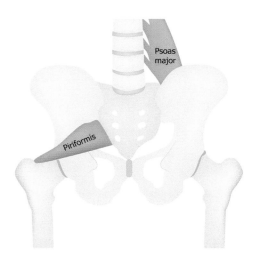

All of these muscles are prone to tension, and when that happens, because of where they are situated and the size of them, they can cause big problems. One of these problems is sciatica. Sciatica can be caused by compression of the sciatic nerve. The sciatic nerve is the largest nerve in the body and runs from the lower spine, through the bottom, down the thigh and into the foot.

When the nerve becomes compressed you can feel pain in various places, such as in your lower back, down your leg or in your foot. If you have acute sciatica, you will know about it. The muscles go into spasm and the pain can be intolerable. Standing, sitting, walking, sleeping all go out the window. You don't know what to do with yourself and everything you do becomes difficult and painful. This is why it's so important to keep these main muscles loose and functioning to their maximum potential.

I had sciatica in my thirties due to degenerative discs, and I wouldn't wish that on anybody. I couldn't walk for six months and at one time thought I would have to give up on my career. What saved me and got me back to doing what I love was exercise and stretching. Gentle exercise to keep my muscles loose and core work to make sure I always maintain a neutral spine. At the age of 30, I was told by a consultant that I had the spine of an octogenarian. The discs in my lower back were all deteriorating, which had compressed the nerves in my spine. I was a mess, but I recovered and now can live a relatively pain-free life, providing I do my exercises and maintain good posture. If time gets the better of me and I fail to do them, I know about it. It's all about perseverance.

The sciatic nerve

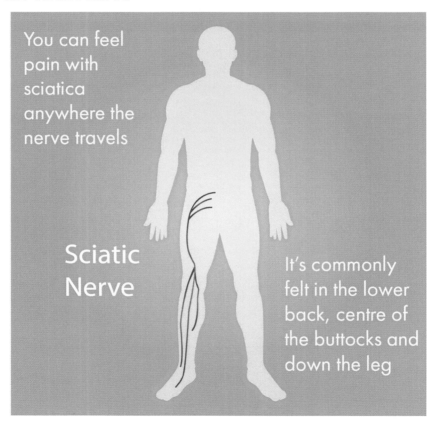

You can feel pain with sciatica anywhere the nerve travels

Sciatic Nerve

It's commonly felt in the lower back, centre of the buttocks and down the leg

The iliopsoas

The iliopsoas loves to be too tight, too short and overstretched. When this happens, it can give you both hip and lower back pain.

The job of the iliopsoas is to lift your knee when you walk and keep you upright. Like most of the important muscles, if you spend too much time sitting, the muscles shorten and problems begin. The muscles can shorten and knot up so much that just stretching won't help. Because of the size and strength of this muscle, when it's fully tensed up it will affect your ability to stand straight.

If you force it, it can make the problems much worse.

Let's do a test to see what condition your muscles are in.

- ▶ Stand with your back against a wall.
- ▶ Lift one leg, bringing your knee to the height of your hip. If you can do that, try holding it there for 30 seconds.
- ▶ Repeat with the other leg, again seeing if you can hold for 30 seconds.
- ▶ If you are struggling to hold your leg then don't force it. Stretch it as shown next and try again.

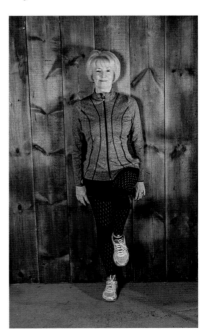

Iliopsoas stretch

- Lie on your back on your bed with your knees bent, hanging off the edge.
- Pull one knee up to your chest while keeping the other thigh flat on the bed. Feel a little stretch in your lower tummy and hold it for 10 seconds.

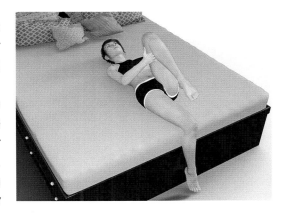

- If all feels ok, repeat on the other side.

Now go back to the wall and try to bring your knee up again. Does it feel any better? Did the knee go up any easier? Can you hold your leg up for longer?

If the answer is no and the stretch did not cause you any pain, try to hold the stretch again, this time for 20 seconds.

There are a few different options to stretch the iliopsoas but I have given you this one as it's the safest stretch to do. As the muscles are so deep and can cause so many problems, it's best to start slowly and persevere. Keep stretching and lifting your knee to check for any improvement.

You are aiming to be able to lift and hold your leg for 30 seconds with minimal effort. When you can do that, you know that the iliopsoas is working well and you can continue with the next exercises without the fear of pulling something and making matters worse.

Muscles of the bottom

The glutes

The gluteal muscles (glutes) are a set of three muscles in your bottom. One of them, the gluteus maximus, is the largest muscle in the body. It's so important to keep these muscles active and strong as they help to control and support so many movements in your body.

If the glutes don't function correctly then your body develops habits to compensate. If your bottom is not strong enough to support you and the load your body creates, the force will end up somewhere else, on muscles that are not built to cope with it. This creates imbalances, stress and tension elsewhere in your body.

It's very important to keep your glutes loose. As you can imagine, if the largest muscle in your body becomes tight, it will have a massive effect on your movement and ability to function correctly.

The glute stretch

As these muscles are so powerful, the last thing you want to do is go in too hard, cause a spasm and make yourself worse. Let's start with a light stretch and then progress.

▶ Lie on your back with your knees bent, feet flat on the floor.
▶ Let your head and shoulders rest on the floor to anchor your body. If this is uncomfortable to do and you find yourself putting a strain on your neck, place a pillow under your head for support.
▶ Now place your right ankle on your left knee. Use your left

hand to keep your ankle in position and, with your right hand on the outside of your right knee, gently pull your knee across your body.

► Don't force the movement, and try to keep the rest of your body relaxed with a neutral spine.

► Hold this stretch for 20 seconds and feel it.

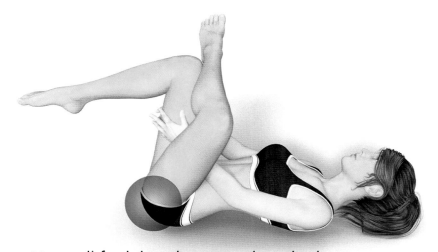

You will feel the glute stretch in the large superficial muscles of your bottom

Where can you feel the stretch? Is it a stretch or is it actually painful? Can you feel it where you are supposed to or are you feeling it elsewhere? How far did your knee travel?

If it felt ok and there was good movement, repeat on the other side. If this felt ok, we will progress; but if it was tight with little movement then don't rush into the next stage until you are happy with this stretch.

➲ Glute stretch 1

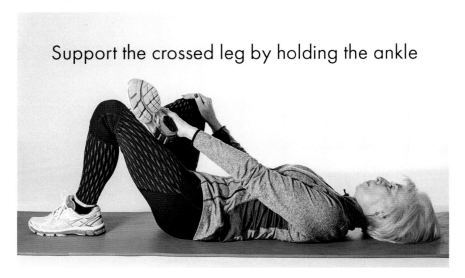

Support the crossed leg by holding the ankle

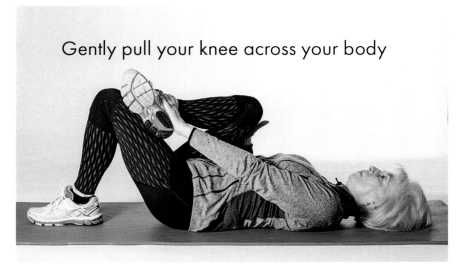

Gently pull your knee across your body

Let's now try a more dynamic glute stretch. Remember, you are now working a massive muscle group. If it doesn't feel ok, that's because it's not. Don't force it. I can't stress enough how much damage you can do to yourself if you ignore the signs your body gives you and try to power through. Gently does it!

- ▶ As before, lie on your back with your right ankle on your left knee, keeping your shoulders down. Relax and breathe.
- ▶ Using both arms, place your hands behind your left leg, just under your knee, and gently pull your leg towards your chest. Try to keep the angle of your left knee around 90 degrees. You are aiming for the left knee to be above your navel.
- ▶ Don't force it, and hold the stretch for 20 seconds.

The stretch should feel a lot stronger and obvious than the previous glute stretch. You should feel it only in the glute. If you can feel it anywhere else, stop. It may be that tight muscles elsewhere are inhibiting the stretch and need to be stretched themselves before you can progress.

You may not be physically able to take hold of your knee with both hands because of complications elsewhere in your body. If this is the case, place a towel around your leg and pull on the towel to bring your leg towards your chest.

If the muscle feels painful or like it's going to cramp or spasm, stop. Give it some time and go back to it later. There is no rush. I want you to do this stretch only if you can feel the muscles easing into it and if it feels comfortable.

If you are straining, shouting out and the vein on your forehead is making an appearance, then you are not ready for this one or you are trying too hard. Ease into it, and with perseverance the stretch will get easier. Don't try to do it all at once. Take your leg to where it feels comfortable and try to improve on it a little each time.

➲ Glute stretch 2

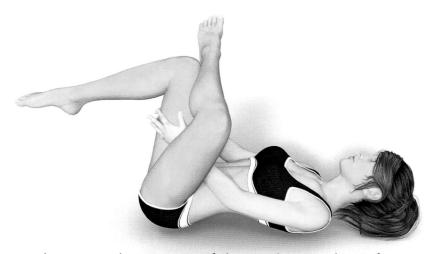

These are big, powerful muscles so don't force it too much but ease into the stretch

8

The leg muscles

The muscles in the front of your thigh are called the quadriceps or quads, and the muscles at the back of your thigh are the hamstrings. Most people will have some sort of imbalance in both sets of muscles, which can lead to hip, knee and back pain. Tight quads can affect your posture, so it's important to keep them stretched and not counteract all the good work that you are doing maintaining a neutral spine and activating your core.

If your quads are tight, they can pull the front of your pelvis down. This will put a strain on your back or weaken your hamstrings, which will also pull on your back. When the quads get really tight, they pull on the hip bone, which tips the pelvis out of position. This in turn tightens the sacroiliac joint, tilts the pelvis forward and pulls on the lower back. This results in an increase in the arch of your lower back making it difficult to maintain a neutral spine, and giving you bad posture. If the front of the pelvis tilts down then the back will tilt up. This puts pressure on the hamstrings and eventually weakens them. The quads overpower the hamstrings, so the hamstrings let the back of the pelvis rise instead of working with the quads to keep it in place. To avoid this tug of war between the muscles in your legs, all you have to do is keep your muscles stretched and active.

The quadricep stretch

Avoid this stretch if you have had a knee replacement.

You will need a tea towel for this stretch.

- ▶ Lie on your front. Take the tea towel and place it around your right ankle.
- ▶ Keep your head down so as not to strain your neck.
- ▶ Using your right arm, pull the tea towel towards your bottom, bending your knee.
- ▶ Keep your knees touching each other and your chest down on the floor.
- ▶ When you can feel a stretch in the front of your thigh and you can't pull any more, gently push your hips into the floor. This will intensify the stretch and you should feel a strong pull in your quads.
- ▶ Hold the stretch for 20 seconds.
- ▶ Repeat on the other side.

The aim is to get your foot as near to your bottom as possible.

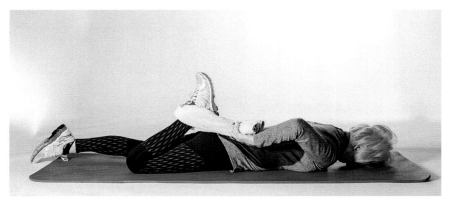

The hamstring muscles

The hamstrings are a set of three muscles in the back of your thigh. They attach in the lower half of your bottom down to behind the back of your knee. The job of the hamstring is to bend your knee and move your hip backwards. Tight hamstrings can lead to lower back tension and vice versa. The more you sit, the tighter your hamstrings become. Sitting can give you a bad back! Tight hamstrings will just add more unnecessary tension to your lower back, inhibit your ability to bend forward and affect the ease with which you can walk. They are muscles that are easy to stretch, with a dramatic effect on your day-to-day living. Let's try two stretches for your hamstrings, one to assess how they are now and the other to mark your progress.

Hamstring stretch 1

▶ First of all, lie on your back, feet flat on the floor with your knees bent.
▶ Maintaining a neutral spine, lower your right leg so it's flat on the floor. Keep your core muscles activated and breathe in.
▶ As you exhale, gently raise your right leg off the floor to a position that feels natural. Don't force it, and try to keep the rest of your body relaxed.
▶ Hold the stretch for 20 to 30 seconds and feel the muscles easing off.

For now it doesn't matter if your leg is straight; your muscles will tell you how far and how much you can stretch. Listen to them. If you can feel a massive pull in the back of your leg or it's shaking then that is enough. If there is hardly any sensation then try placing your hands behind your knee and gently pull the leg with your hands, increasing the stretch.

➲ Hamstring stretch 1

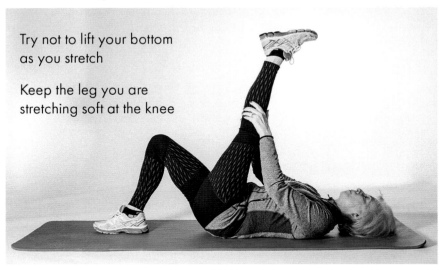

Try not to lift your bottom as you stretch

Keep the leg you are stretching soft at the knee

The most important thing to remember is that the leg not being stretched stays at 45 degrees bent at the knee. Tight hamstrings have a direct impact on your back so, if done incorrectly, this stretch can hinder as much as it can help. Lying down with both legs out straight will arch your back and take away your neutral spine. If your hamstrings are particularly tight and you try to stretch without a bent knee on the supporting leg, it's all too easy to pull or even tear a muscle, causing quite a lot of damage. If done gently and slowly, paying attention to what your body is telling you, and easing into your tight muscles, this stretch will have a dramatic effect on your body. Looser hamstrings will help you to bend over and make it easier putting on your socks and shoes, taking the strain off your lower back and glutes.

Providing this stretch is done with a neutral spine, is not forced and is taken gently, it's a good indicator of what condition your hamstrings are in. A good stretch is being able to take your leg straight up with ease so it sits vertically from the floor. If you can do this then let's move on to the next stretch. If not, keep working on it until you are comfortable and stretching feels natural.

Hamstring stretch 2

Whereas the first hamstring stretch isolated your hamstring muscle, this stretch will use a few more muscles. Only attempt it if you felt ok doing the previous stretch, as now you will be progressing the stretch. As well as targeting your hamstrings, you will be working your back and arms. If you are carrying too much tension in any of these places, one will play up against the other, putting too much of a strain somewhere else, and you will not effectively stretch the hamstring itself.

To do this stretch, you will need a rolled-up tea towel. Start by sitting down with both legs straight in front of you. You will feel a natural strain on your lower back. To avoid this, bend the knee of one leg (the leg you are not stretching). Put it in a position that feels comfortable. It doesn't matter too much if it's not vertical, but the stretch will be more comfortable if you can pull it towards your chest so that the leg can fall away gently to the side. A bent knee will give you a neutral spine, taking away the pull in your back and making the stretch more beneficial.

► Place a rolled-up towel under your straight leg. This will stop you overstretching the muscle. It keeps your knee soft and limits the stretch going into your calf muscle, which would inhibit its effectiveness in the hamstring.
► Gently stretch both hands towards your toes, moving as far down your leg as possible without overdoing it.
► You should feel a pull in the back of your leg where you are stretching the muscle. The further down your leg you take

your hands, the more you will feel the stretch. Stay within your comfort zone. Don't stretch so hard that it becomes painful, but also don't make the stretch too light.

► When you are happy with the amount of stretch and it feels engaged but comfortable, think about what is happening with your arms and back. Try to stay relaxed when holding the pose.

► Feel the muscles lengthening in your arms, back and leg, and hold the stretch for 20 seconds.

► Then, gently ease your muscles off and sit back up.

How far down your leg did you manage to get your hands? I would be happy with anywhere between the top of your socks to your toes. Between your knee and your socks needs work, and past your toes is excellent!

Now, repeat the stretch with the other leg.

➲ Hamstring stretch 2

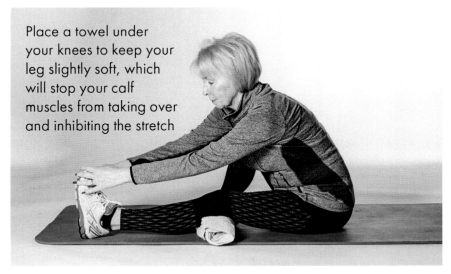

Place a towel under your knees to keep your leg slightly soft, which will stop your calf muscles from taking over and inhibiting the stretch

9

Putting together a routine

Now we have covered the basics, let's put some of it together.

For any of this to work and actually start changing your day-to-day life, you need consistency. Just a little. By doing a bit of exercise each day, your muscles will start to feel looser.

Exercise needs to be consistent because just doing a bit every now and then doesn't give your body a chance to change. Your muscles will just tighten up and, in the exercise gap, revert to how they were. Consistency gives your muscles a chance. A chance to lengthen, tone and produce the results that you are hoping for.

I want you to do this routine daily. Make it part of your day just as much as cleaning your teeth or showering is. If you do this, you will notice results and it won't take long to do so.

As you did earlier on in the book, start your routine with a gentle walk. You are just walking to warm up your muscles so you don't have to walk for a long time. About 10 minutes is plenty. As before, remember your checklist:

- ▸ Maintain a neutral spine.
- ▸ Gently activate your core.
- ▸ Open your chest and relax your shoulders.
- ▸ Swing your arms.
- ▸ Walk heel to toe.
- ▸ Take deep, regular breaths, in through your nose and out through your mouth.

Try to keep this checklist in mind throughout your walk, staying relaxed as you go, and not trying too hard.

As soon as you get back, you will stretch. It's beneficial to stretch straight after exercise to get the most out of your muscles being warmer and more flexible. Also, as you exercise, the muscle fibres shorten so a stretch at the end will lengthen them again and stop them becoming any tighter.

Make sure you hold each stretch for at least 20 seconds. Any less will not lengthen the muscle fibres, and too long can cause injury by stressing them.

Do the following stretches after your walk for 20 seconds each.

- ▸ Chest stretch
- ▸ Hug the tree stretch
- ▸ Cat stretch
- ▸ Quad stretch
- ▸ Hamstring stretch (1 or 2)
- ▸ Legs down to one side stretch
- ▸ Glute stretch (1 or 2)

➲ Stretches after a walk

Hold all stretches for 20 seconds

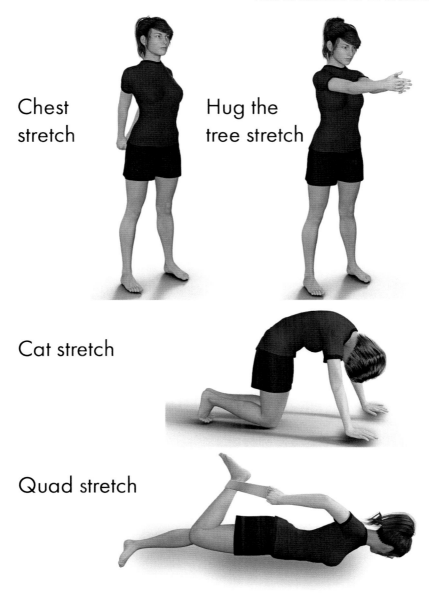

Chest
stretch

Hug the
tree stretch

Cat stretch

Quad stretch

59

➲ Stretches after a walk

Hold all stretches for 20 seconds

Hamstring stretch

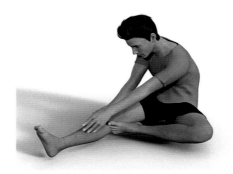

Legs down one side

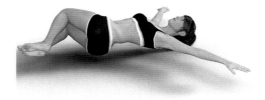

Glute stretch

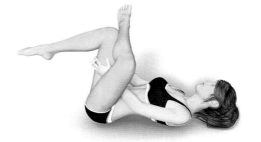

10

Strength training

Strength training will make your muscles stronger, increase bone density and help with balance and coordination. As I mentioned earlier in the book, with age your muscles weaken, which causes imbalance between the groups of muscles, fatigue and injury. I believe that, to get the best result, there is no point in starting to strengthen your muscles until they are ready. That means until they are loose, as relaxed as you can get them and with minimal imbalances. If you start training your muscles when they are tight, and with incorrect posture, all you are doing is strengthening the weaknesses, adding to the imbalances and causing more pain.

This is why I am covering the strengthening exercises now and not before. I want you to do this next section only when you are confident to do so and feel you are ready to move on from the exercises earlier in the book. Remember, there is no rush. Better to go slow and steady than end up causing yourself more pain and discomfort.

If you feel you have achieved all the goals in the stretching sessions of the book and are now content with the way your body performs, it's time to move on. Let's build a better you!

You will use two types of exercise for strength training: compound and isolation. Compound exercises use more than muscle, often getting groups of muscles to work together, whereas isolation exercises target a specific muscle. Let's start with the isolation exercises as they are less complicated and easier to do well.

The exercises begin at your feet and work up. You can do the first one either standing or sitting. Do one leg at a time. The aim is to loosen off your ankle and see if there are any hidden surprises there!

➲ Plantar and dorsiflexion

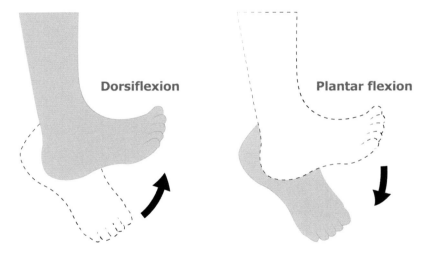

Dorsiflexion   Plantar flexion

▶ Point your toes away from you (plantarflex), holding for a second, then point your toes towards you (dorsiflex) and hold.
▶ Repeat 10 times on each foot.

As your toes travel towards you, your calf muscles (in the back of your leg between your ankle and knee) will tighten. How much your foot moves depends on the amount of tension stored in your calf. The looser your calf, the more movement you will have in your foot.

▶ Next rotate your foot at the ankle 10 times in one direction and then 10 times in the other.

Was that a nice smooth action with no restriction and full range, or was it sore, clicky or staggering with hesitation? In order to seek out knots and deal with tension, look for hesitation. If your muscles are absolutely fine there won't be any. It's imbalance, weakness and tension that cause hesitation by putting stress on the way the muscles move. Your muscles end up fighting against what should be a natural action, causing hesitation.

Calf raises

▶ Stand at arm's distance from a wall with your palms flat on the wall at shoulder height.
▶ Your feet should be hip distance apart, your heels and toes parallel.
▶ Engage your core and breathe in. As you exhale, push off your heels and rise onto your toes and hold for a second, then come back down.
▶ Try to keep the pressure in the balls of your feet. You don't want to push up too high and end up with too much pressure on your toes.
▶ Don't rush, but ease up and down, holding for a second at the top. Repeat 10 times.

Try to keep your feet square when you rise. Quite often, because of problems elsewhere, the heels start moving inwards, or the feet roll out or in. That will not work the muscle fibres in your calf evenly, resulting in an imbalance.

Calf stretch

As you have just worked your calf muscle, shortening the muscle fibres, you now need to stretch them out to lengthen them again.

- ▶ Using the wall for support, place both palms onto the wall and stand with your feet hip distance apart.
- ▶ Take a step back with one leg, as far as it can go with your heel pressed firmly into the floor.
- ▶ Lean forward into the thigh of your other leg. Make sure both feet are facing straight forward and keep your back heel glued to the floor.
- ▶ Hold the stretch for 20 seconds. Repeat with the other leg.

⮑ Calf raise and calf stretch

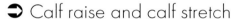

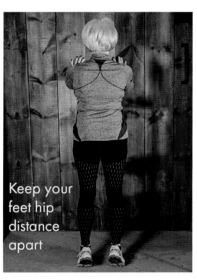
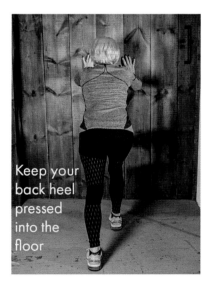

The calf is a strong, tough muscle so don't be worried if the stretch feels strong. The bigger the muscle, the stronger the stretch. Just remember that you are stretching not tearing. There is a fine line between a strong stretch and pain. Try not to cross over into the pain zone as it's easy to damage the muscle by tearing it.

The bridge

This exercise strengthens your hamstrings. Lie on an exercise mat if you have one, or a thick towel or blanket.

► Lie on your back with your knees bent, feet hip distance apart and arms by your sides.
► Take in a few deep breaths, relaxing your upper body. Engage your core and, maintaining a neutral spine, breathe in.
► As you exhale, use your core and bottom muscles to lift your bottom off the floor, placing your body weight onto your shoulder blades.

You will feel a pull on the muscles at the back of your thigh. If you feel anything stronger than a pull, like the muscles beginning to cramp, gently lower yourself down and stretch your hamstrings again. You should aim to hold the bridge for 30 seconds without dropping your bottom and keeping your core engaged and spine neutral.

➲ The bridge

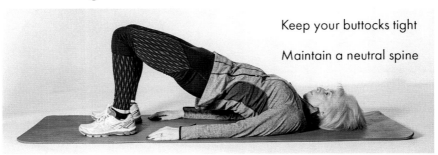

Keep your buttocks tight

Maintain a neutral spine

Hamstring stretch

- ▶ As before sit on the floor with your legs out in front of you.
- ▶ Roll up a towel and place it under your left knee.
- ▶ Take your right foot and place it on the inside of your left knee. If you can, let your right knee fall down towards the floor.
- ▶ Slide both hands down your left leg towards your left foot.
- ▶ When you feel a strong stretch, hold for 20 seconds.
- ▶ Repeat on the other side.

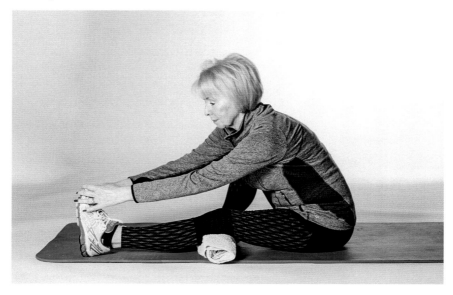

The clam

This exercise will isolate the gluteus medius, one of the three main muscles in your bottom. I have included an exercise for this muscle as it's one that I am always treating. When you stand, your weight is evenly distributed over both feet. When you walk, however, it's not. The gluteus medius supports your pelvis from falling on the other side when you lift your leg.

I come across many clients who have weak glutes that are not functioning correctly, resulting in an imbalance in the hip and a tight gluteus medius. This upsets the muscles in the bottom and eventually can lead to the muscles becoming so tight that they clamp down onto the sciatic nerve.

Basically, a happy gluteus medius means that you will walk in the way your body is meant to. Your muscles will stay active and loose.

▶ Lie on your side with a pillow or your underneath arm supporting your head. You can place a thin cushion or towel under your hip too if it's painful to lie on your side.
▶ Start with your legs, hips and shoulders in a straight line.
▶ Bend your knees so that your lower legs are at a 90-degree angle to your body. Make sure your knees don't move, keeping them in line with your chest.
▶ Making sure you have a neutral spine and your core is activated, tilt your hips slightly forward. If you don't do this, as you begin the exercise, your back will try to take over and you will lose alignment.
▶ Keep your feet glued together and lift your top knee. Then slowly lower it back to the start position. Only go as far as you can keeping your core on and maintaining alignment.

The movement should be small as you are trying to isolate the gluteus medius. You should feel it just behind your hip in the top section of your bottom. It should feel difficult to execute and is certainly not an easy exercise to master.

If it feels easy, and your knee is flying up and down, then your back has taken over, you've lost your core and you are not isolating the correct muscle. This should be a slow and controlled exercise that feels difficult to perform with the correct technique. To achieve the technique is a massive step in becoming a core master! Do this exercise 10 times then repeat on the other side.

➲ The clam

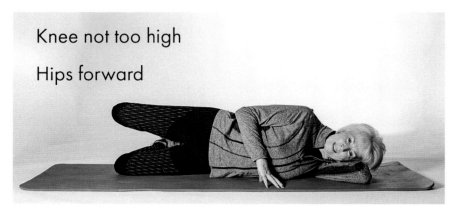

Knee not too high

Hips forward

The most important thing to remember with this exercise is the position of your hips: the further forward the better; too far the other way and you will use your back. If you can lift your knee higher than your shoulder you are not targeting the correct muscle.

Gluteus medius stretch

Avoid this stretch if you have had a hip replacement.

This is the best stretch to target the gluteus medius as it doesn't put pressure on your spine. If your body allows it, you will feel the stretch radiating from your bottom into your lower back. However, for this stretch to be beneficial, everything else has to be working correctly. Quite often, the muscles in the legs, back and bottom are too tight and can inhibit this stretch. Wear and tear in the hip also restricts this stretch. If that's the case you will feel it in your groin, not where you are meant to.

Give it a go, but if you can feel it anywhere other than where you are meant to, stop and do the glute stretch you learned earlier in the book. It doesn't isolate the gluteus medius, but it's better than not stretching at all.

- ▶ Lie on your back with your left leg straight. Lift your right foot across your left leg and place it on the outside of your left knee, with the sole of your right foot pointing towards your body, not flat on the floor.
- ▶ Gently anchor your body with your right shoulder and place your left hand on your right knee.
- ▶ Gently pull your right knee to the floor, not too hard, turning your pelvis. As soon as you feel a stretch, stop and hold for 20 seconds. Repeat on the other side.

Your knee should never touch the floor. It doesn't have to move much to get the stretch. If you try too hard there is a good chance of setting off another muscle somewhere else, causing an unwanted spasm. Less is more with this one!

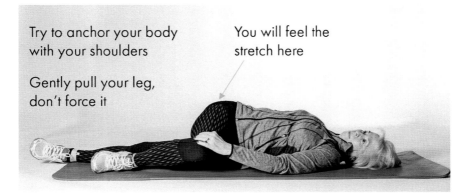

Try to anchor your body with your shoulders

You will feel the stretch here

Gently pull your leg, don't force it

Single leg raise

This is another one of my favourite exercises because it's so effective. I hardly ever massage anyone who has even balance in their quads, and this exercise goes a long way to achieving that. As I touched on earlier, having uneven quads puts pressure on your hips, back and knees resulting in pain due to imbalance.

You did the basic version of this exercise before. Now, let's push it a bit further. You will need a rolled-up towel.

The midline of the thigh

Before you do this exercise, you need to learn about the midline, which is an imaginary line passing straight down the centre of the thigh.

Imagine drawing a line down the centre of your leg. Start at the top of your thigh, go down the centre of your thigh, pass through the centre of your knee and continue down into your middle toe.

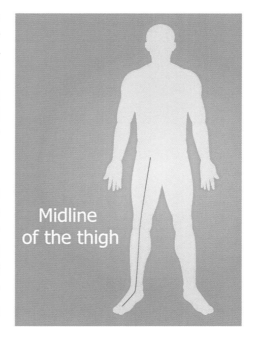

You need to visualise the midline for this exercise to make sure that your four quad muscles are worked evenly. If the midline is off then they won't be. If your toes are facing away from your body you will instead isolate your inner thigh muscles, and if your toes are facing towards your body, you will work the outside of your thigh. As you are striving for balance in the thigh, you need to keep your toes central and feet facing forward.

▶ Lie on your back with your knees bent, feet flat on the floor.
▶ Straighten one leg and place the rolled-up towel under that knee. You do this to make sure you don't overextend your knee, which will pull the muscles behind it.
▶ In order to maintain a neutral spine, the leg you are not using should stay bent at a 45-degree angle, with your foot flat on the floor. This helps to stop you arching your back as you raise your leg.
▶ Keep your hands by your side and make sure your neck is comfortable.
▶ Using your straight leg, tilt your toes towards your body to activate the calf and lock your leg.
▶ Make sure your leg is in the correct position using the imaginary midline. Activate your core.
▶ Breathe in and, as you exhale, raise your leg off the floor a few centimetres.
▶ Hold it there for 10 seconds, checking that the midline is still correct and remembering to breathe.
▶ Then gently lower your leg.
▶ Repeat 5 to 10 times with the same leg (depending on how much your body can cope with).
▶ Then do the whole sequence with the other leg.

Remember not to arch your back, and keep checking your core is on. Don't overdo it. This exercise is just as much about being able to maintain your core as about lifting your leg in the air.

➲ Single leg raise

Point your toe towards your face to lock the leg; this activates the calf muscle

Activate your core and keep your upper body relaxed

The leg not being used stays bent to help maintain a neutral spine

11

Compound exercises

Now it's time to put everything you have learnt together and get your body working in harmony. Let's start with the most difficult exercise first, the chair squat. This exercise will work pretty much every muscle in your body and, if done correctly, is a massive achievement.

Chair squat

First of all, you need to find the correct chair. Remember earlier? The height of the chair is just as important as the exercise itself. When sitting, your bottom should be level with or slightly higher than your knees. Place the chair next to a wall so that it can't slip backwards during this exercise.

▶ Start standing in front of the chair, a few centimetres away from it – just enough so that the backs of your legs are not touching the chair.
▶ Soften your knees and open your chest.
▶ Activate your core and make sure your spine is neutral. Place your hands by your sides at chest level with your elbows bent. Keep your eyes facing forward, fixed on something in front of you.

- With your feet hip distance apart, toes very slightly facing out, sit down on the chair by pushing your bottom back and pushing your hands forward until your arms are straight.
- As soon as your bottom touches the chair, stand back up, bringing your hands back to your chest and bending your elbows.
- Repeat the whole action 10 times.

Make sure your eyes stay looking forward and you don't look down. Also, be aware of what your knees are doing. It's absolutely normal for your body to try to cheat. This usually happens with your knees moving towards each other. It's a normal habit in which your mind is telling your body that you are better off doing so. Be aware of this and keep your knees equal distance apart throughout the entire exercise.

Make sure that your knees don't travel forward past your toes. By keeping them just over your ankles and pushing your bottom back, you will really engage your quads and gluteus muscles, keeping unwanted pressure out of your knees.

➲ Chair squat

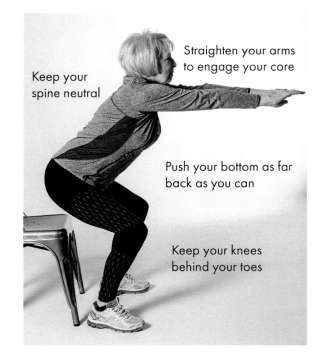

Straighten your arms to engage your core

Keep your spine neutral

Push your bottom as far back as you can

Keep your knees behind your toes

Knee raise to waist

It's best to do this exercise holding onto something solid. I always suggest the kitchen worktop.

- Stand side on to the worktop and put your inside hand palm down for support. Stand tall, eyes forward, with an open chest and relaxed shoulders. Place your feet hip distance apart and remember the midline on both thighs.
- Slowly, using the outside leg raise your knee to waist height, keeping the angle of your knee at 90 degrees. Your back will want to arch so don't let it. Keep your core activated and your spine neutral.
- When your knee is up to your waist, hold it there for 10 seconds, breathing and focusing on your core.
- Do this knee raise 10 times, holding for 10 seconds each time, and then repeat with the other leg.

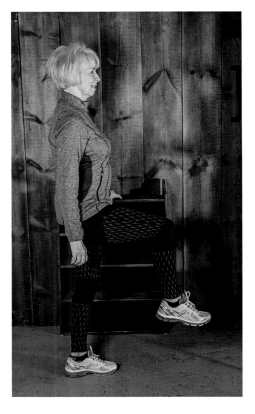

With this exercise you are getting your thighs and hip working together, which will dramatically help with walking and making sure your pelvis stays in the correct position.

➲ Knee raise to waist

Stretches

▶ Knees fall down to one side stretch
▶ Glute stretch
▶ Gluteus medius stretch
▶ Quad stretch

Box press-ups

I will give you three versions of this exercise that increase in difficulty. Use the first version if you have difficulty kneeling or can't get onto your knees.

Box press-up 1

Place your hands, shoulder distance apart, onto the edge of a kitchen worktop with your palms on the edge and fingers on top.

▶ Keeping your hands where they are, step back one foot at a time, making sure you can keep your heels down on the floor. Keep your heels, knees, hips, shoulders and head in alignment. Activate your core and tighten your bottom.
▶ In one complete motion, keeping that alignment, lower your body towards the work surface by bending at the elbows. Stop when your elbows reach a 90-degree angle and pause for a second.
▶ Feel your chest muscles engage and use them to push yourself back to the starting position.
▶ Repeat 10 times.

Try not to rely just on your arms and shoulders for the push-up phase of the exercise. Work on being able to feel it in your chest muscles as much as your arms and shoulders.

➲ Box press-up 1

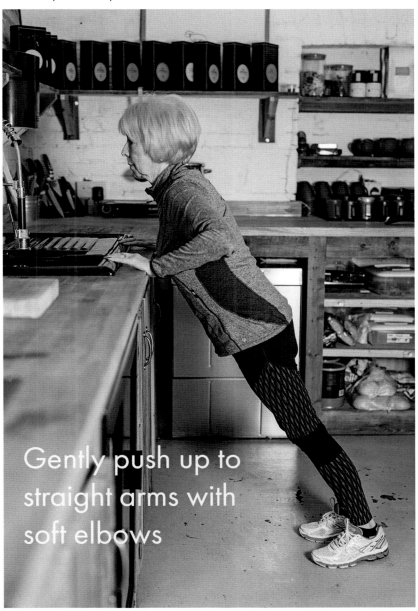

Gently push up to straight arms with soft elbows

➲ Box press-up 2

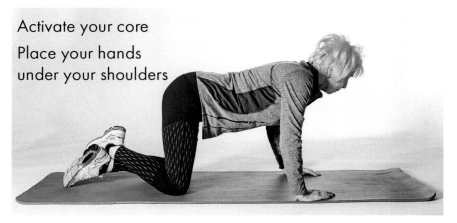

Activate your core
Place your hands under your shoulders

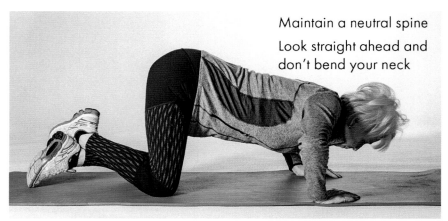

Maintain a neutral spine
Look straight ahead and don't bend your neck

Box press-up 2

▸ On all fours on a mat or towel, place your knees slightly apart and your hands shoulder distance apart directly under your shoulders.
▸ Make sure your hands and knees are parallel, not rotated.
▸ Cross your ankles and take your feet off the floor. Align your bottom and your head, keeping your eyes looking straight

ahead. Try not to look down as this will put a strain on your neck.

▶ Activate your core and lower your chest towards the floor by bending your elbows until they reach a 90-degree angle.
▶ Pause for a second and then use your chest muscles to push yourself back up to the starting position.
▶ Repeat 10 times.

During the exercise, keep a neutral spine to avoid arching or hollowing your back. Keep your thighs at 90 degrees to the floor and don't push your bottom backwards.

Box press-up 3

▶ Lie on your front, cross your ankles and lift your feet off the floor by bending from the knees. Place your hands either side of your body, palms down just below your shoulders.
▶ Straighten your head and neck and find a neutral spine. Engage your core and tighten your bottom.
▶ Breathe in and, as you exhale, push yourself off the floor until your arms are straight.
▶ At the top, pause for a second and then slowly lower yourself back down to the starting position.
▶ Repeat 10 times.

Make sure your elbows stay facing each other and keep them slightly soft, not locked, at the top position. You don't want to overextend your elbows or start rotating your shoulders, and soft elbows will avoid this.

You will find this exercise much more difficult than the previous two simply because it uses a lot more body weight. The hardest thing here is keeping a neutral spine throughout the exercise.

On the way up, the natural reaction is to hollow your back, lifting your shoulders out of alignment; and on the way down, your back will try to arch. Keep everything straight from your knees to your head. It's difficult to achieve, and if you find it too much, stay on exercise 2 until you have the strength or confidence to progress to this one.

➲ Box press-up 3

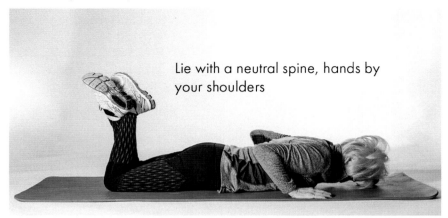

Lie with a neutral spine, hands by your shoulders

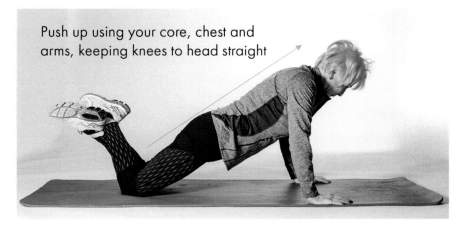

Push up using your core, chest and arms, keeping knees to head straight

Stretches

Triceps stretch

- ▸ Stand tall in a relaxed position with a neutral spine.
- ▸ Raise your left arm straight up and bend the elbow, placing your left arm below your neck, palm on the middle of your upper back.
- ▸ Take your right hand and place it on top of your left elbow. With your right hand, gently push down on your left elbow so that your left hand slides down your back.
- ▸ Stop when you feel the back of your left arm stretching and hold for 20 seconds.
- ▸ Repeat with the other arm.

When doing this stretch, don't lean or tilt your body. Keep it in alignment, with a neutral spine and strong core.

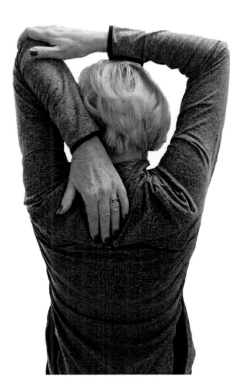

Shoulder stretch

- ► Stand tall in a relaxed position with a neutral spine.
- ► Straighten your left arm and place it across your body parallel to the floor.
- ► Put your right hand on your left arm between the shoulder and elbow and pull towards your chest.
- ► Keep your elbow the same height as your shoulder, and as soon as you feel a stretch, hold for 20 seconds.
- ► Repeat with the other arm.

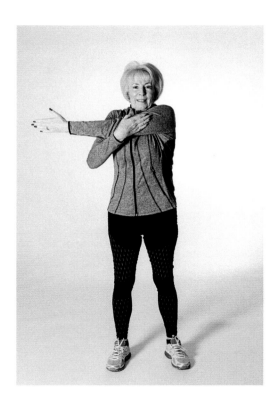

Chest stretch

- ▸ Stand tall with a neutral spine, feet hip distance apart. Open your chest and relax your shoulders. Activate your core.
- ▸ With straight arms, interlock your fingers behind you. Push your arms up while pulling your shoulder blades together.
- ▸ Stop and hold the stretch when you feel your chest stretching and your arms will not go up any further.
- ▸ Hold for 20 seconds, taking in big breaths. Breathe in through your nose and out through your mouth. Keep your eyes forward, trying not to bend your neck.

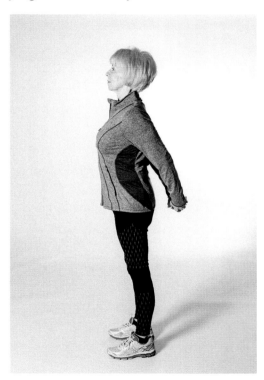

The plank

The plank is one of the best exercises you can do. Not only does it target your core but it will also make a huge improvement to muscles all over your body. When performing a plank, you hold yourself through your arms, shoulders, back, bottom and legs, so all these muscles are being strengthened and developed.

It's an isometric exercise. The benefit of an isometric exercise, especially the plank, which uses so many muscles, is that joint and muscle length don't change. This means the exercise is static, with no moving parts, so you limit injury on the joints and muscles.

► Start on the floor on all fours.
► Place you forearms on the floor with your elbows directly under your shoulders. Your elbows should be at a 90-degree angle and your hands shoulder width apart.
► One at a time, place your feet back so that your legs are straight and off the floor. Hold a straight line from your heels through to your head, eyes looking at the floor.
► Activate your core and hold the plank for 10 seconds.

If you are struggling to keep a neutral spine or you can feel it in your back, all you need to do is raise your bottom a little higher, taking the arch out of your spine.

If 10 seconds feels ok then try 20 seconds. The optimum is 30 seconds. Any more than that and your core will tire, making your hips drop and placing your body weight into your back as it begins to arch.

➲ The plank

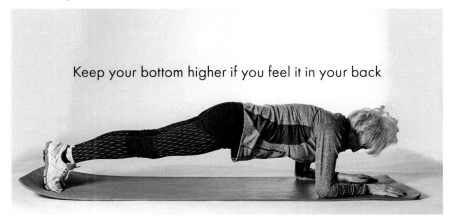

Keep your bottom higher if you feel it in your back

When you have finished, hold a cat stretch for 20 seconds.

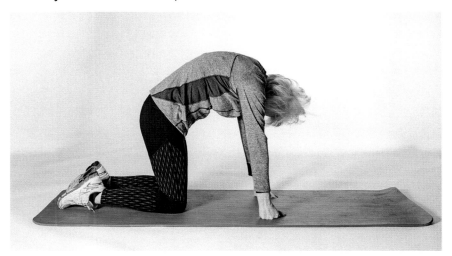

12

Getting you moving

Now that you have a strong core and have woken up your muscles, let's add a little aerobic exercise to get the blood pumping around your body. These exercises will improve your balance, coordination and strength and will work out your heart and lungs a little. I am going to keep it simple and focus on five exercises. I am adding a bit of movement to tie everything you have learnt together and make you more active and mobile.

Side steps

If your balance is not the best then do this exercise holding onto the kitchen worktop. If you're confident and solid on your feet then do it without holding on.

▶ Stand tall with a neutral spine, relaxed shoulders, open chest and feet hip distance apart.
▶ Take your right leg and step out to the side.
▶ Now bring your left leg towards your right, back to hip distance apart.
▶ Take four steps like this over to the right: so, right leg, left leg, right leg, left leg and repeat.
▶ Then take four steps travelling to the left.

Never have your feet closer than hip distance apart. The closer your feet, the less balanced you will be so the more chance you'll have of falling. Try to keep your arms from being too static, and if you feel comfortable doing so, add in a little arm movement as you travel.

Do this exercise for one minute, catch your breath and then move on to the next exercise.

➲ Side steps

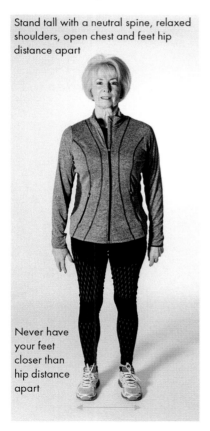

Stand tall with a neutral spine, relaxed shoulders, open chest and feet hip distance apart

Never have your feet closer than hip distance apart

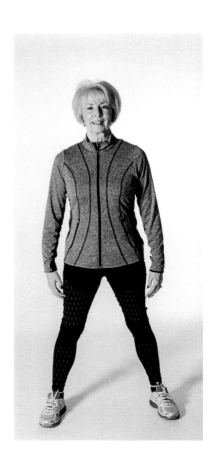

Marching on the spot

▶ Stand tall, feet hip distance apart, open your chest and relax your shoulders.
▶ Activate your core and, with a neutral spine, start marching on the spot.

Keep your eyes up as looking down will make you top heavy and a lot more likely to fall. Bring your knees no higher that hip height because any further will arch your back.

Keep your elbows at 90 degrees and swing your arms from the shoulders.

Do this for one minute then move on to the next exercise.

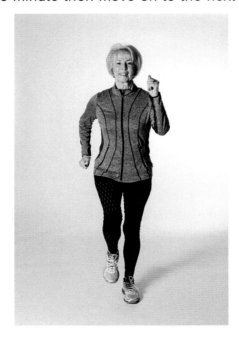

Hamstring curls

► Stand tall, feet hip distance apart, open your chest and place your hands on your hips.
► Activate your core and, with a neutral spine, bend one leg back from the knee, bringing your heel towards your bottom.
► As soon as you can't go any further, place your leg back down and repeat with the other leg. Keep this action going for one minute: heel to bum, heel to bum...

If you have the confidence and feel secure on your feet then add in some arms. Keeping your elbows bent, as each heel goes back, swing both elbows back to match.

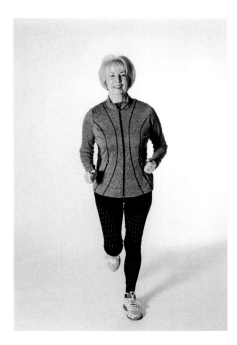

Heels forward bicep curls

▸ Stand tall, feet hip distance apart, open your chest and place your hands by your side, elbows in.

▸ Activate your core and, with a neutral spine, place your right foot forward, tapping your heel on the floor, and bring it back.

▸ Repeat with your left foot then carry on tapping your heels forward with alternating feet.

▸ When you have your rhythm, add in bicep curls. Using both arms at the same time, from a straight position, bend your elbows, bringing your hands towards your chest and trying to keep your elbows close to your ribs.

Keep tapping your heels and curling your arms for one minute.

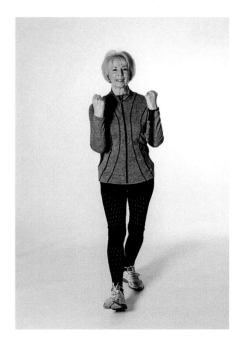

Kick back with hands forward

▶ Stand tall, feet hip distance apart, open your chest and place your hands on your hips.
▶ Activate your core and, with a neutral spine, place your right leg behind you and touch the floor with your toes, then bring the leg back and repeat with your left.
▶ Keep alternating your feet and, when you have the rhythm, bring your hands up to your chest with bent elbows. With each step back, reach forward with both arms in a pushing motion.

Keep your arms at shoulder height and bring them back at the same time each foot goes back towards your body. Legs out, arms forward. Legs back, arms in.

Keep that going for one minute.

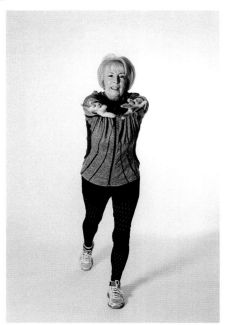

Putting it all together as a routine

Now let's do a little five-minute routine. Remember, work within your capabilities. If you feel pain or dizzy then stop and have a rest. Make sure you drink some water after the routine to rehydrate. Muscles don't work properly when they are dehydrated.

March on the spot	1 minute
Side steps	30 seconds
Hamstring curls	30 seconds
Side steps	30 seconds
Hamstring curls	30 seconds
Kick back reach forward	1 minute
Hamstring curls	1 minute

Now stretch all the muscles you have just used. Hold each stretch for 20 seconds, taking nice big breaths.

► Chest stretch
► Shoulder stretch
► Triceps stretch
► Calf stretch
► Cat stretch
► Quad stretch
► Hamstring stretch
► Glute stretch

13

A few exercise routines to get you under way

Programme 1

Stand with back against wall	Hold for 1 minute
Chest stretch	Hold for 20 seconds
Shoulder shrugs	10 repetitions
Hug the tree stretch	Hold for 20 seconds
Tea towel pulls	10 repetitions
Shoulder stretch	Hold for 20 seconds
Chin to chest stretch	Hold for 20 seconds

Programme 2

Marching on the spot	1 minute
Chair squats	10 repetitions
Hamstring curls	1 minute
Chair squats	10 repetitions

Side steps	1 minute
Knee raises	10 on each side
Cat stretch	Hold for 20 seconds
Glute stretch	Hold for 20 seconds each side
Quad stretch	Hold for 20 seconds each side

Programme 3

Door hinge	10 on each side
Legs down to one side	Hold for 20 seconds each side
Single leg raise, bent knee	8 on each side
Bridge	Hold for 3 sets of 20 seconds
Plank	Hold for 30 seconds
Cat stretch	Hold for 20 seconds
Hamstring stretch	Hold for 20 seconds each side

Programme 4

Cat stretch	Hold for 20 seconds
Box press-ups	2 sets of 10 repetitions
Superman	10 on each side
Windscreen wipers	5 on each side
Iliopsoas stretch	Hold for 20 seconds each side
Glute stretch	Hold for 20 seconds each side
Gluteus medius stretch	Hold for 20 seconds each side
Quad stretch	Hold for 20 seconds each side

Programme 5

Calf raises	10 repetitions
Calf stretch	Hold for 20 seconds each side
The clam	10 repetitions each side
Glute stretch	Hold for 20 seconds each side
Plank	Hold for 30 seconds
Cat stretch	Hold for 20 seconds
Door hinge	10 on each side

Something to think about!

Diaphragmatic breathing

Diaphragmatic or belly breathing is a useful technique to add to your repertoire. It will strengthen your diaphragm, help you relax by lowering stress levels (it can lower cortisol, the stress hormone), lower your heart rate, help lower blood pressure and help with back pain.

Belly breathing is great for when you have had 'one of those days' and just need a few minutes to yourself to unwind. The technique is simple and straightforward to master. You can do it sitting or lying down.

▶ Lie on the floor or sit in a comfortable upright chair, knees bent and with a neutral spine.
▶ Place one hand on your chest and the other on your stomach.
▶ Breathe in through your nose, letting your belly expand up and out. Try to limit any movement in your chest and focus it into your stomach. Use your hands to feel the movement in both your chest and stomach.
▶ Breathe out through your mouth, pulling your belly back in.

I always breathe in and out to the count of 3 as that suits me, but you may feel happier with a 2 or 4 count. Repeat for a few minutes.

➲ Movement of the diaphragm

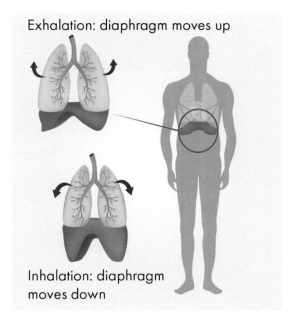

Exhalation: diaphragm moves up

Inhalation: diaphragm moves down

Now over to you

Now to the business end of changing your life. You have taken the first step and bought this book. You have gone to all the trouble and effort of reading it and doing the exercises. Please don't stop there. Keep on and be consistent. Just a little something every day will dramatically change your life.

I have started you off with five programmes to get you under way, but they are not set in stone. It's up to you how you exercise, but use this book as a reference for technique and posture. Mix the exercises up, but do something every day, be it stretching or strengthening.

The one thing I want from you is that you walk every day with your core on. Walk and listen to your body. Feel what is going on and deal with it. The routines can be done as you wish, but obviously, the more you do, the stronger and fitter you will become.

All that is left to say is good luck rebuilding a better you. Don't stop. With a little effort and perseverance, you will get there.

For more information, please visit johnmolyneux.com